Chapter 1.

We had an accident.

My name is Betty! This is my true life story, in August 2018 as I was walking towards where to take an auto bus back to my house, was so tired sitting at the local clinic in my city at Alessandria, Italy. where I have resident , I was 6 month pregnant, after doing OGTT test , I was so tired and hungry, as the bus arrived, I entered and sat down so relaxed, we were 6 people with the driver in the bus, we pass through children hospital, we turn at the back of the stadium, we turn towards Zona Orti , there was another bus who wanted to turn , our bus was still going forward faster, this company bus came out so quickly, the driver was trying to come out from where he packed, the company driver hit our bus while on a full speed , I saw glasses of our bus window entered into the eyes of a woman, another man was injured, I hit my stomach on an iron, I was in pain and I was scared at the same time , they took me to the hospital with an ambulance, i didn't knew this was just the beginning, the pain was un describing, they gave me drips and pain relieved since I was pregnant they can't allow me to do an resonance, after 5 days I was discharge from the hospital, it happened to me towards mid August 2018, in September 2018 I was in pain , my husband called an ambulance again to take me to the hospital, I was given again 2 drips again for 4 days, I couldn't walk, when I try to take a little walk, I will be in tears, many called me lazy, some of my husband friends called me names, I was once told that some Africa women who are pregnant they go to farm to cultivate till the day they give birth to their children, they were too naive to see and remember that I had an accident with pregnancy, am an Africa woman but I have health issues.

I felt a little bit better and I was hiding some little pain I was experiencing, because I was really tired of going back to the hospital, so I pretended that I was perfectly fine, one midnight, I couldn't sleep, my husband had to call an ambulance again in October 2018, I was given drips again to relieved the pain, no one knew what I was facing, some of the nurse were so angry when they see me in the hospital, they gossip in silent, while some will call me by my surname to make jokes that I loved to stay in the hospital, I was worried about my baby, I was always praying to God to make us both survive this pregnancy, in November 2018 I went to the hospital for a normal check up, I was told the blood test I did was not alright, the doctors admitted me, I was again in the hospital, when every Nurses, some of the Doctors saw me , they were so surprised again to see me , my families were so scared that I will not survive it, I looked so tired , when I walked or stroll I was always in pain , I don't know what was wrong with me , I have other 2 children back home in Nigeria before living for Europe, when I was pregnant with them , I gave birth to them normally without no complications, I understand I had an accident but the hospital said I was fine but what was happening to me , I don't know , the doctors too can't explain my pain but I was admitted due to they saw that I have Gut but is due to digestion disorder, but the pain is unexplainable said the doctors, I was given drips everyday, morning and night, I was in the hospital for 2 weeks and I beg them to allow me go home, they refuse at first but with much pleading, they decided I should go but if there's a problem I should come quickly, I replied okay I will.

I went home happy, when I arrived home my husband has already cooked before he came to pick me up at the hospital, I bathed and eat, I watched some Nollywood movies which newly came out, then I slept off. That night I was in pain, the pain was so much that I can't sleep, I was crying with pain, my husband couldn't sleep too, we managed the whole situation, but I was so sorry for my husband because the next day he will go to work, the next day came, my husband had to call his employer that he can't come to work due to my health issues.

The day I was given to come to the hospital came so I went, I arrived at the hospital with my luggage and the luggage of my baby, I and my husband was so happy, that night my husband went home because I need to still stay for another 3 days to do some blood test before the labour day, the first night I spent in the hospital I had a dream, I saw some gathering of people pushing me into a pit and another white woman brought out, then I woke up, I prayed that God should save me and this time I was now scared, so scared that I couldn't eat.

That morning the nurse came to fix a drip for me, the nurse asked how excited I was to be ready give birth, I told her that finally I will be free from all pain and everything that is happening to me.

Chapter 2.

My things was stolen in the hospital.

I was so press, I needed to use the restroom, the lady in my room was called by the nurse to come to the labour room, I was now alone in the room, the sisters of the lady in my room came to ask about her then I explain where she is to her sister, she left immediately to meet her sister, after she left I had to go to the bathroom with the drip on my hand, I walk through the passage to the near by restroom, my room has no restroom, I left my phone under the pillow case, my bag and my wallet too, so I quickly went to the restroom, I finally finish my business there, as I was coming from the restroom, I saw a man coming out from the room where I was in the hospital, I said to myself in mind thank God the lady just gave birth may be that was while she has many visitors, I enter my room, I sat on my bed, as I was reaching out to where I left my phone, it wasn't there I scattered the whole bed , no where to be found , I reached out to where my bag is, my wallet was missing, my documents, debit card and some cash was stolen including my passport, I rang the emergency bell , one of the assistants nurse came , my husband came at that point , then I explain to them that as I was coming back from the toilet , a man was coming out of my room , I taught it was the husband of the other lady but I was wrong, they called police immediately, the ask us to follow them , we walked pass through many wards until we reach their office at redcross, we lay complaints, nothing was refund or done about it, my money, phones, wallet ATM was gone within a twinkle of an eye.

My Advise to Every one going to the hospital to be admitted, or visit, please if your room has no toilet and you need to walk to where the toilet is, please take your personal belonging like phone, wallet, e.t.c , take them with you to the restroom, shine your eyes, your hospital room mate might be thieve, anyone can walk in at any time pretending to be visiting, be at alert.

 I entered back in my ward , the next day was the day that I will give birth but I was so angry that nothing was done , I was given only the copy of the complaint papers, I started thinking about that have happened to me and the poor baby in my stomach, at this time I was s scared, I don't know what else to expect or possibly go wrong, I started praying again that God should help me give birth safely, I started feeling lonely, imagine staying in a country where there is no family, Benjamin who is a family friend has done a lot for us, he always try to cheer me up, he always brought me food, things, so that I can feel better, even one or two times my husband gave Benjamin keys to our apartment to bring things for me while my husband stay with me, he is more as a family to us, when he heard about what had happened to me, he came, he stay for 2/3 hours ,he told me he had things to do then he left, I was ready for tomorrow, it was my big day , I talked to him on the phone, and the nurse came to instruct me about the next day, she told me a lot about the gel insertion , I asked her about the advantages and disadvantage, she replied, it has no disadvantage, then she fix the drip and then she left. I was relieved, I had joy rolling through me then again I was scared I don't know why , I knew something was not alright but I don't know what that was , I started praying, after praying I slept off, about 21:00 to 22:00 , a nurse came to ask how I was feeling, I replied fine , even if I was not , I was tired to complain every time, so I slept back.

The next day on November 27th 2018 I waked up so early, every body that knew me knows I always wake up so early, even if I don't have anything to do, I always wakeup early .

Chapter 3.

The labour day.

I prayed while on the hospital bed, After praying I tried to get up from the bed despite the pain , my husband was not with me , he had to go home to prepare the nursery, clean the house and everything, we were alone at this moment, I reached out for my language to take out clean cloths and new things to wear , I was still having that feeling of fear and joy , I went to the bathroom to bathed and change my clothes, after putting on a beautiful floral maternity dress, I put on some body spray to smell nice , I return back to my room at the hospital to wait for the doctors and nurses to call me for the gel insertion, I was feeling worried, but joy was rolling back again, anytime I felt worried or fear in my heart , at the end joy always come , I think that is the confirmation of the Holy spirit making joy rolling in my hearts, they holy spirit never leave his beloved ones, the holy spirit was telling me to calm, he is with me always. At 9am they called me for the insertion, I was so happy, I have never felt happier since I was pregnant, I went with the nurse to the labour room, I taught I will stay in the labour room after the insertion, but I was told to go back to my room, then my husband was waiting for me, we talked about what he did at home, I told my husband about the insertion, he asked, how are you feeling right now, I said I was feeling like before nothing has changed so far, my husband sat on a chair, then I climb on my bed to relax but I couldn't, the pain was increasing, my husband was supporting me, at 12pm I couldn't sit, I couldn't eat anything, the contraction is unexplainable, I have had 2 children before but this one is different, at 17:00 I was crying bitterly, we called the nurse, they came, I was examined, I asked her how is it , she said I was in 5cm dilated, I replied only , 5cm dilated, please don't let me die like this, my husband snap in, you won't die, the nurse went, I continued to pray and hoping to overcome and triumph, my husband couldn't eat or leave me , he never stop praying too or having faith, Benjamin wanted to come , we said he shouldn't come until I give birth so that he can see his niece, at 19:00 my husband couldn't take it again, he had to call the nurses to do something, I was taken to the labour room, I was there in pain and also hope the pain end sooner after I gave birth, my husband was by my side.

At 21:00 one of the hospital nurse came the doctor to examine me, they also fix epidural at my back, I wasn't feeling any pain while they put the Epidural at my back, I remember someone told me that it's painful but in my case, I was not feeling any pain, the doctor if the baby sac breaks by it self or they do it for me, then I replied, they do it for me, so they went, the nurse came to do the Artificial rupture of membranes for me , because I was 10cm dilated, after they left.

At 22:00 I started feeling strange, my hands was shaking and my eyes , I was feeling dizzy, my said I passed out , I was hearing a far distant calling , then I regain consciousness because I remember I asked my husband why are shouting my name and shaking me like that with a silent voice, they were nurses, doctors all round me.

I was transferred quickly to another bed, as they were talking me away from the labour room, I was not feeling any contractions any more , I was feeling weak , tired, I was feeling as if I was sleeping, the last word I said was please save my daughter, save her.

Chapter 4.

I was rushed to the operation room.

My husband said he waited outside, he was not allow to enter the emergency room, After 1 hour, he heard the cry of our beautiful daughter Michelle, some minute later the light of the hospital off then it turns on back immediately.

A doctor came to give my husband good and bad news, he was told that I was given birth but they don't know why I have not wake up, my husband started hitting the walls of the hospital angrily, he said to them I have been complaining and admitted every month in this hospital, didn't you doctors see what I was going through, my husband called Benjamin, some of close family and friends but only Benjamin was there with my husband at the hospital, my husband saw doctors, nurses running to the emergency room where I was , my husband said at this point he was confused, desperate, he called his brother and family in Nigeria to raise their voices in prayers for me, Benjamin called his mother to pray for me, my husband was calling my name to not go, he was talking as if I was there with him , my husband was not allow to see me , after some hours , they brought me out on the bed with oxygen on my nose, they told my husband they are talking me to the ICU, he followed them when they got there, they told my husband to stay outside to wait.

After 1 hour they came they gave my husband a paper to fill, he collected the papers and requested to see me, my husband said when he saw me, I have 7 types of machine saving my life, they sew 1 on my hand, 1 on my neck, 1 that go from my nose to my throat, Electrocardiogram on my chest, blood infusion going on, drips on the other hand, oxygen on my nose, he busted in tears, he was talking to my body as if I was listening to him, this time make sure his faith is firmed, he put all his trust in God, he couldn't break the news to my family, then they ask him to go out to wait for their call.

Benjamin took my husband home, my husband busted to tears , our neighbours at that time was peculiar and Family, peculiar ask my husband how I was doing ?, my husband explained everything to her and her family, she said because of the news she couldn't celebrate her birthday, but my husband speaks to her she shouldn't worry, she should go on with her celebration.

Benjamin cooked for my husband to eat , he was there for me and my family, even if we are not related by blood , I call him my brother, A friend in need is a friend indeed.

People tried to speculate lies about Benjamin being a fornicator, he sleeps with people's wife, girlfriends, if he is that kind of person I would have know, Benjamin has been with us ever since as a family friend and a brother, I don't care about the lies they speculate about him, he will still be my brother, he has not done it to me so I will never believe it, let them say , I don't care .

Benjamin is always disappointed when he heard about people confronting him to accuse him of the lies people fabricate against him. Trust me , he is a good person, Benjamin has a place in our home and heart always, even if the whole word turn their back at him , I and my family will never do that, people ask us why am I so close to

Benjamin, I replied to them, imagine someone who stood by us in bad times, is not only our friend any more, he is a family, a brother from another mother.

My husband started speaking to his pastor in Nigeria, my pastor too, every one of them were praying for me to be heal, the doctors didn't tell my husband what wrong, they had to do series of test, but I was receiving treatment, my husband went back to the hospital the next day, he was praying and thanking God in faith, he was believing that I should wake up, a doctor told my husband that if I did not open my eyes my husband should forget about me, my husband replied with faith, she will wakeup.

My went to the children ward to visit Michelle, he took her in his harm, she is so beautiful, he changes her clothes, diapers and feed her, the children ward doctors were asking how was doing, my husband was crying, each time they ask of me, he will reply with tears, he was so happy to see Michelle but at the same sad, he was so scared that if something eventually happens, people will call him bad head, or he used me for ritual, things like that happens in African.

Chapter 5.

My waking up from coma

Is as if I was dreaming, I don't even know what happened to me , I saw my self in a wide place, some people were farming in a wide big long land , which some people were passing through a tin Road, they were in white, they were matching in accord, they were having white hairs, white beard , the ones at the back that I saw were men , I don't know if women were among them, I walked pass through those ones in labour, I was rushing to meet up with those one on the tiny road, the last man on the line spoke to me, go back your time is not now, go back, I was so stubborn, I don't want to go back, despite where they were passing was narrow, I don't even care , I remember I have regret going with them, I was happy but then again I heard some people shouting my name from afar , I remember a light was drawing me back from this lovely people that i wanted to follow, the light was so bright that can blind someone eye's, I couldn't see through those light , I deemed my eyes, then I wanted to open my eyes, it was so heavy, I couldn't raise my hands , my legs, even my body is so heavy, I tried to open my eyes, but heavy , my legs and hands was not still working, the little I could open was as if i was still in that brighter light, I saw my husband, doctors, nurses, all round me , I couldn't speak, I was whispering to try to ask my husband , where was my baby.

I was so thirsty, I asked for water, the nurses said it's not possible, they can't give me water to drink , every time I opened my eyes am always seeing nurse, doctors, all around me. The nurses did not leave my side , I saw doctors and nurses from pregnancy wards, they came to visit me , they were all awesome, if I was in my country, I would have died, but God did not only love me he gave second chance to leave to declare his words, I know I was not perfect but his mercy endures forever.

I was taken to intensive therapy, I still have on oxygen, Electrocardiogram on my chest, I was taken care of like a baby, I was not allow to stand up from the bed, one morning I ask them to let me see my baby, 2 of the nurses at the pregnancy ward came with Michelle, I saw Michelle for the first time, I was so happy, I felt joy in my heart, the joy rolling in my heart was unbelievable and I was tearing, Michelle was so small and beautiful, people came to great her, nurses, doctors, Oss, they congratulate us, the nurse left with Michelle, when my husband left, I started thinking about children without their mother, how are they doing without their parents or mother especially, I was thankful to God to allow see My daughter and my

2 boys in Nigeria on video, God really saved me, the next day I decided I will start leaving my life to the fullest, I requested to dress up , they clean me up gauze and soap, they wear me my clothes, then after they left , I sat down on my bed, I started practicing how to get up on my bed , they came suddenly that I shouldn't, they I sat back on my bed, I was so determined , I was thinking that if I don't help my self no one will, I was ready and scared that maybe my legs are no more walking, I wanted to feel the floor again while walking.

The next day before anyone could come , I come down from my bed , I turn then hold the iron of the bed , at this time I said to my self , no backing down, I will not give up, I stay there I couldn't walk or move normally, when the nurses came they remove the oxygen, and the Electrocardiogram, then they gave me a chair and helped me to sit , I sat, they arrange my bed and after they left, I started walking, by holding the iron of my bed, I felt good , happy , I said to myself that this is a complete testimony, they after some minute, I started I remove I hands from the iron little by little, I started drawing my leg on the floor to move it and it worked. I worked throughout the passage like 3 time and I was so tired, the next day I requested that I wanted to stay close to my child , they agreed, I was transferred to pregnancy wards , 2 OSS came to take me on a wheel chair and I was tearing with joy, I was so grateful as we arrived at the pregnancy ward. The Oss take me to the nurse in charge of admissions, they took me to a room with bathroom and I settled in.

Chapter 6.

I arrived at the pregnancy ward.

I requested them bring my baby, after some minute they brought Michelle to my room, my husband came, my Italians mama came, they brought things for me, I couldn't still be able to eat , I always eat liquid because I couldn't swallow properly, my throat was painful and I was coughing badly, I asked why am I coughing, they told me that due to the drip they pass through my nose to my throat, that is why I was coughing, after they left, I told my husband to change Michelle clothes and wipe her face and body with some wipes, people came to visit me, peculiar came to visit too.

The next day, the doctors came to ask how I was doing I said I felt much better than before, I ask If I can take my bath, they said yes, my husband took my daughter Michelle to the children ward, he then came to prepared to bath, I bathed the blood on my body off properly and I felt so relieved, how awful to not bathed for almost 2 weeks after given birth, I felt so good after talking my bath and after dressing up, my husband took me back to my bed, in the evening my husband left , I was now with Michelle, my breast milk was not rushing, Michelle was hungry, I had to call the children ward nurses to bring Michelle food, Michelle was crying so much that I had to call them to help me , I couldn't do anything, I couldn't carry her for so long , they came to ask if they should take her back, I said yes for her wellbeing but I felt sad that I couldn't take care of her well , it wasn't my fault, if I wasn't in that condition, I will have taken care of Michelle by my self, the next day I told the doctors that I wanted to go home, they check the test they did for me to see how I was doing, they said they will let me know, at 12pm on that day, they called me to come to the doctors office, I went, they cut off the stitch on my stomach, they cut it, one by one, it was so painful, after they finished cutting it, I was taken to TAO centre to register I was told I had pulmonary Embolism that was why I was in Coma, I was lucky to survive this, more than 60,000 die of this illness in a year, most of those who die, do so with in 30 to 60 minutes after symptoms start, in 25 percent of people who experience pulmonary embolism (PE), the first symptoms is sudden death, I was given Claxane 6000 to take 2 times a day, then every week I was going to TAO centre for blood test and control, it got to a time my hands, stomach every where in my body where I was given my self this injection was now painful, I requested for oral medicine, they agreed to change my medication to Coumadin . I was taken this medication for 1 year and also going for control too, my baby Michelle is now 4 years old but she has some health complications, thank God for every thing, I believe when there is life, there is hope, it is only God who is capable to do miracle like this, no one can.

www.ingramcontent.com/pod-product-compliance
Lightning Source LLC
Chambersburg PA
CBHW080438220526
45465CB00009B/3334